YOUR KNOWLEDGE HAS VALUE

- We will publish your bachelor's and master's thesis, essays and papers

- Your own eBook and book - sold worldwide in all relevant shops

- Earn money with each sale

Upload your text at www.GRIN.com
and publish for free

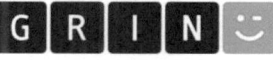

Bibliographic information published by the German National Library:

The German National Library lists this publication in the National Bibliography; detailed bibliographic data are available on the Internet at http://dnb.dnb.de .

This book is copyright material and must not be copied, reproduced, transferred, distributed, leased, licensed or publicly performed or used in any way except as specifically permitted in writing by the publishers, as allowed under the terms and conditions under which it was purchased or as strictly permitted by applicable copyright law. Any unauthorized distribution or use of this text may be a direct infringement of the author s and publisher s rights and those responsible may be liable in law accordingly.

Imprint:

Copyright © 2016 GRIN Verlag, Open Publishing GmbH
Print and binding: Books on Demand GmbH, Norderstedt Germany
ISBN: 9783668592179

This book at GRIN:

http://www.grin.com/en/e-book/381240/diabetes-in-qatar-an-overview

Patrick Kimuyu

Diabetes in Qatar. An Overview

GRIN - Your knowledge has value

Since its foundation in 1998, GRIN has specialized in publishing academic texts by students, college teachers and other academics as e-book and printed book. The website www.grin.com is an ideal platform for presenting term papers, final papers, scientific essays, dissertations and specialist books.

Visit us on the internet:

http://www.grin.com/

http://www.facebook.com/grincom

http://www.twitter.com/grin_com

Diabetes in Qatar

Name: Patrick K. Kimuyu

Introduction 2
Overview of Diabetes 3
Causes of Diabetes and its Related Social Determinants of Health................................. 3
Pathological Impacts of Diabetes... 6
Diagnosis of Diabetes in Qatar 7
Diabetes Treatment and Management 7
Levels of Prevention and Health Promotion 8
Healthy Public Policy in Qatar 8
Recommendations 9
Conclusion 9
References 11

Introduction

Diabetes in Qatar has seemingly become an enormous challenge to public healthcare systems. Qatar is one of the GCC countries which are known to have the highest diabetes incidence rates. In a global ranking, Qatar is ranked six whereas the United Arab Emirates and Saudi Arabia who are members of the GCC countries are ranked second and third, respectively in regard to incidence rates of diabetes (Dwevedi & Goyal, 2010).

Current epidemiological reports indicate that an estimated 16 percent of the adult population in Qatar is suffering from diabetes, in which type 2 diabetes is the most prevalent compared to type 1 diabetes. However, other clinical reports indicate that diabetes prevalence among children below the age of five years in Qatar has also assumed upward trends. For instance, prevalence rate for diabetes among children was reported to be 13.7% in 1997, but this rate has more than doubled to reach 28.2% in 2007 (Dwevedi & Goyal, 2010).

From an epidemiological perspective, the burden of diabetes to Qatar's healthcare system seems to be overwhelming. Therefore, it has become a significant concern in community health nursing because the number of Qatari diabetic patients seeking for medical treatment has increased significantly. This situation has been worsened by the rising trends of obesity prevalence rates. Currently, 45% of the population in Qatar is obese in which 55% of diabetic patients are obese (ANSA, 2013). Therefore, this correlation in incidence and prevalence rates of the two diseases complicates prevention and health promotion measures in Qatar. As a result, Qatar's efforts to reduce the prevalence of diabetes have been faced with enormous challenges. However, the country is optimistic that the Qatar Diabetes Project and Stem Cell Projects will be successful.

In regard to the risk factors, the unprecedented increase of diabetes prevalence is attributable to lifestyle and genetic factors. Clinical studies reveal that most people in Qatar have changed their cultural lifestyle to western-related lifestyle, and this is believed to have contributed significantly to the current diabetes crisis. However, genetic factors have also been found to have contributed to the high prevalence rates.

In general, diabetes issue in Qatar needs appropriate epidemiological measures to reduce its burden to the country's healthcare system in which social health determinants and epidemiological indicators will help in addressing the issue. Therefore, this research paper will provide an overview of diabetes in Qatar.

Overview of Diabetes

Diabetes mellitus is a metabolic health condition which is characterized by increased blood glucose, a condition referred to as hyperglycemia. It is popularly known as diabetes. There are two forms of diabetes: Type 1 diabetes (Insulin-dependent Diabetes) and Type 2 diabetes (Insulin-independent Diabetes). Type 1 diabetes is also known as Juvenile or childhood diabetes because it occurs during childhood and persists into adulthood (CDC, 2010). In contrast, type 2 diabetes occurs during adulthood; therefore, it is referred to as Adulthood diabetes.

Diabetes is believed to occur due to absence or insufficient production of Insulin by the β-cells of the Islets of Langerhans located in the pancreas. Insulin is a hormone which is responsible for the regulation of glucose in the blood circulation. Type 1 diabetes occurs due to genetic disorders that cause defects in the pancreas or in the Insulin receptors that are located on the surface of body cells (Masharani, 2008). On the other hand, Type 2 diabetes occurs due to Insulin resistance by the body cells.

Causes of Diabetes and its Related Social Determinants of Health

Diabetes is caused by high calorie intake especially carbohydrates. Research shows that consumption of high amounts of simple sugars such glucose lead to increase in blood glucose. High levels of glucose in the blood circulation after a heavy meal trigger the production of insulin from the β-cells of the Islets of Langerhans. Insulin is released into the blood circulation and then it gets transported to the body muscles, where it binds with the insulin receptors that are located on the surface of the body cells. Binding of insulin to the insulin receptors triggers a signal transduction in the intracellular region of the body cells, leading to the opening of glucose channels on the cell membrane (Coddington & Hisnanick, 2001). Glucose enters into the body cells where it is oxidized to generate chemical energy.

Excessive stimulation of the pancreas to release insulin leads to production of high amounts of insulin, which in turn, causes insulin resistance by the body cells. This condition is referred to as glucose intolerance because body cells do not take up glucose from the blood circulation. Therefore, glucose accumulates in the circulation leading to energy deficiency in the body cells.

Diabetes affects all the body cells especially the active muscle cells that are usually involved in generation of ATP energy in the body (Brandt & Churchill, 2003). However, its signs and symptoms are manifested in the kidneys, eyes and the circulatory system. It also affects the brain, the nervous system and the heart.

It has been found out that most causes of diabetes are influenced by several social determinants of health which have led to the increase of the prevalence rates in Qatar. Ordinarily, diabetes and the other non-communicable diseases are caused by socially determined behaviors and lifestyles. For instance, nutritional paradox such as eating habits and tobacco smoking are some of the contributing factors to the increased prevalence of diabetes among the Qatari population.

Some of the most significant social health determinants which are believed to have caused the prevalence rates of diabetes in Qatar include unhealthy environments, lack of social protection, lack of universal primary healthcare, challenges of childhood development and low literacy level.

Qatar and the other GCC nations have been experiencing challenges in designing efficient strategies to ensure childhood development enhances disease control. As a result, most children in Qatar are not protected against childhood diseases. This is probably the reason as to why prevalence trends of diabetes seem to have increased significantly among the young generation.

The second social determinant of health, which seems to have contributed significantly to the increase in diabetes prevalence in Qatar is unhealthy environments (Siddiqi & Watts, 2008). Qatar is one of the fast growing countries in the Middle East, in which oil resources have led to the emergence of rural urban centers. As a result, a large percentage of the national population has migrated to the urban centers where community health is relatively compromised by the growth of slums. It has been reported that slums are increasing rapidly in most urban centers in Qatar. Ordinarily, unsafe environment, which is characterized by overcrowding of people in the slums has been found to be one of the most significant factors causing obesity among children and adults. This is so because; slum areas lack adequate space for physical exercise and recreational facilities. Therefore, Qatar's urban population faces a high risk of becoming obese and overweight both of which are predisposing conditions for diabetes.

On the other hand, Qatar is characterized with inefficient employment settings. For instance, youth unemployment in Qatar has been an enormous social and economic challenge. In addition, informal sector employment has also been found to be high in Qatar (Siddiqi & Watts, 2008). As a result, Qatar's population comprises of a high percentage of the low-income population leading to the rapid expansion of slums in urban centers. Epidemiological studies indicate that socio-economic factors are related to the occurrence of obesity and diabetes. Therefore, informal sector employment and unemployment are some of the contributing factors towards the increase of diabetes among the Qatari population.

Moreover, lack of universal primary healthcare has also led to the increase of diabetes case in Qatar. Qatar's healthcare system has been quite unsustainable owing to the scarcity of healthcare resources and services. As a result, out-of-pocket healthcare expenses have become an enormous burden to the Qatari population. It has been found out that most people in Qatar do not receive adequate healthcare services (Siddiqi & Watts, 2008). Therefore, disease screening services are relatively unavailable for patients. Ordinarily, screening for diabetes enhances disease prevention and control strategies. Therefore, the unprecedented lack of screening services in healthcare facilities has compromised prevention approaches, despite the government's efforts to address the issue.

Lack of education is the other social determinant of health which has led to the increase of diabetes in Qatar. It is believed that literacy level in Qatar is relatively low, primarily among women. Ideally, cultural aspects are believed to be the principal causes of low literacy levels among Qatari population. Demographic reports indicate that most women in Qatar are not educated, and empowerment strategies have been fruitless in the last decade. As a result, most women are not employed; thus, they are dependent on their male counterparts causing an economic strain in the nation. It is believed that lack of education among women in Qatar is responsible for high prevalence rates of diabetes because women are more affected than men. However, literacy levels in Qatar are increasing significantly, and this is expected to enhance prevention and control of diabetes.

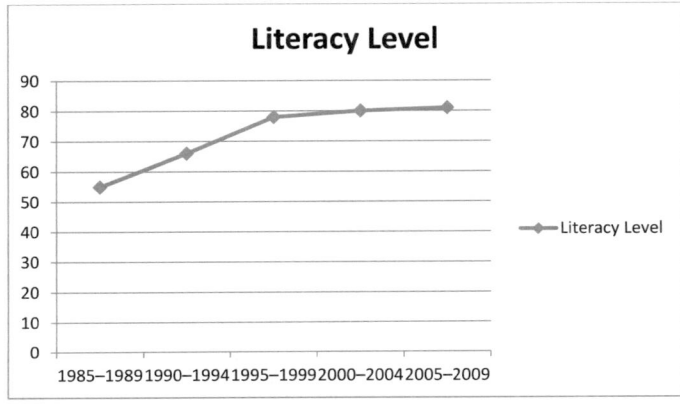

Figure: Literacy rates in Qatar (Siddiqi & Watts, 2008)

Moreover, social exclusion is also believed to have contributed to the increase of prevalence rates of diabetes in Qatar. It is believed that some social groups such as migrants from low-income countries and ethnic groups in Qatar do not access adequate health services. In most cases, ethnicity and social identity lead to the exclusion of these groups. Therefore, lack of opportunities to access healthcare services has contributed to health inequalities in Qatar, and high cases of diabetes serve as ultimate health outcomes.

Pathological Impacts of Diabetes

The principal symptoms of diabetes are polyuria, polydipsia and polyphagia. Polyuria refers to excessive passage of urine. Urine passed by diabetic patients is usually sweet due to the presence of high levels of glucose. Polydipsia is a condition which leads to feeling of thirst because much water in the body is lost through urine. Diabetic patients experience persistent hunger, even after meals because their body cells are glucose deficient, although there is a high level of glucose in the blood circulation. This leads to excessive intake of food, a condition known as polyphagia (Coddington & Hisnanick, 2001). Other symptoms include weight loss, fatigue and blurred vision.

Chronic diabetes causes several fatal impacts especially when treatment is not provided or delayed. Some of the principal impacts of diabetes include blindness, hypertension and stroke. The pathophysiology of these health complications can be explained by digressing into the physiological conditions the cause them.

Health records show that most diabetic patients experience hypertension due to Atherosclerosis. Ordinarily, accumulation of glucose in the blood circulation impairs oxidation of lipids. As a result, triglycerides and cholesterol levels in the blood circulation increase above their reference range. This leads to inefficient transportation of cholesterol by the High Density Lipoprotein (HDL), which is referred to as good cholesterol (Brandt & Churchill, 2003). Synthesis of HDL decreases significantly leading to an unprecedented increase of triglycerides and Low Density Lipoprotein (LDL), also known as bad cholesterol. Consequently, LDL reacts with Reactive Oxygen Species (ROS) to form highly reactive complexes that adhere on the surface of blood vessels. Binding of the reactive complexes with the epithelial cells on the surface of blood vessels leads to the formation of plaques that make the blood vessels inelastic. Further accumulation of reactive complexes on the blood vessel surface leads to a disease condition referred to as Atherosclerosis. This condition is characterized by the stiffening of the blood vessels: thus, interfering with the blood flow. In retrospect, Atherosclerosis causes blockage in small vessels such as blood capillaries; hence generating counter pressure against the cardiac systolic pressure and the ultimate result is hypertension (Masharani, 2008).

Moreover, blockage of blood capillaries leads to the death of body tissues that are supplied with nutrients by the blocked capillaries. This condition is usually fatal when it occurs in the brain because it causes death of some brain cells, leading to stroke (Brandt & Churchill, 2003).

On the other hand, blindness occurs due to accumulation of cholesterol deposits in the cornea. Medical diagnosis shows that most diabetic patients in Qatar have yellowish deposits in the eyes which look like cataracts. Therefore, excessive accumulation of cholesterol deposits in the eyes leads to blindness or blurred vision (Brandt & Churchill, 2003). In addition, blindness can be caused by high blood pressure in the eye region which interferes with impulse conduction of the optic nerves.

Diagnosis of Diabetes in Qatar

In Qatar, diabetes is usually diagnosed through blood sugar tests such as Fasting Blood Sugar (FBS) test and Random Blood Sugar (RBS) test. Normal blood sugar levels ranges between 3.5 to 8.0 mmMol/L. Blood sugar levels beyond this range indicates glucose intolerance and levels beyond 11.0 mmMol/L indicates diabetes. Diabetes can also be diagnosed through biochemical analysis to determine the level of glycated hemoglobin (HbA_{1c}) (Coddington & Hisnanick, 2001).

A population-based study indicates that 10.7% of Qatari population lives with diagnosed diabetes in which Impaired Glucose Tolerance (IGT) accounts for 12.5% of the diagnosed population, whereas Impaired Fasting Glucose (IFG) accounts for 1.3%.

In regard to gender, women are the most affected by diabetes with 53.2% while a low percentage of 46.8% represent Qatari men who are diagnosed with diabetes in the ages of 40 years and above (Bener et al., 2009).

Diabetes Treatment and Management

Unfortunately, diabetes is not curable, but there are various treatment and management approaches. Diabetes management involves the formulation of nutrition schedule to avoid diets that are rich in simple sugars such as refined foods, commonly referred to as fast foods. Health records show that proper diet plays a principal role in preventing disease progression. Research indicates that diabetes can be reversed through a nutritional approach especially during its onset, although research trials are underway to validate this assertion. Physical exercise is also recommended for diabetic patients because it helps to burn excess glucose in the body (CDC, 2010). These approaches have been known to be extremely effective in management of diabetes.

Additionally, diabetes can be treated medically through the use of medicines that enhances glucose uptake by the muscle cells. Treatment of Type 1 diabetes involves intravenous administration of artificial insulin. This supplements the body's insulin production leading normal glucose utilization in the patient's body (Brandt & Churchill, 2003). However, it is worth noting that individuals suffering from Type 1 diabetes are supposed to take daily insulin injections throughout their lives.

Levels of Prevention and Health Promotion

Diabetes has been found to be preventable especially through nutritional approaches and physical exercise. Research indicates that individuals who engage themselves in physical exercise for at least 15 to 30 minutes a day lower the risk of diabetes by 96 percent (CDC, 2010). In addition, adoption of a diet regime that excludes simple sugars has also been found to reduce diabetes risks.

In general, diabetes deaths can be reduced through early diagnosis to prevent progression of the disease condition into chronic stages. People require undergoing regular blood sugar tests to monitor their blood glucose levels (Pompei, 2006). Moreover, diabetes awareness programs will make people informed about diabetes; hence prevention will be easy.

Currently, Qatar has designed a comprehensive health strategy which aims at the prevention of chronic and non-communicable disease including diabetes. For instance, evidence-based programs such as the national screening program and nutrition and physical activity program are designed to address diabetes as one of the high-priority diseases in Qatar.

Healthy Public Policy in Qatar

In regard to public health policy, Qatar is in the process of designing a comprehensive health framework through the establishment of health regulations to address healthcare challenges including the burden caused by diabetes. The Supreme Council of Health has designed several approaches to ensure full healthcare coverage. Some of the most significant regulations include the development of national regulatory framework which is based on safety standards, quality and evidence to enhance the realization of sustainable healthcare through the improvement of health outcomes of the Qatari population. The second regulation is to ensure regulation of healthcare facilities and national health standards for public and private healthcare institutions to prevent the increase of diabetes (Al-Maadheed & Qahtani, 2011). Moreover, Qatar's health policy aims at enhancing patients' advocacy to support patients' rights and complaints.

Recommendations

Ideally, prevention of diabetes and health promotion in Qatar requires several considerations for diabetes prevalence rates to be reduced in the foreseeable future.

First, Qatar requires the establishment of a multi-sectoral approach in fighting diabetes. An ideal strategy will include improving management of diabetes, diseases screening and promotion of healthy dietary regimes. It will also require the incorporation of health risk reduction factors among the Qatari population through enhancing disease awareness and physical activity.

The second approach will comprise of unifying diabetes priorities in the country. This will ensure efficient integration of governmental and non-governmental healthcare agencies to support early-detection, which will play a significant role in reducing morbidity and mortality related to diabetes in Qatar.

Another preventive and control approach, which appear to be relevant in reducing the prevalence of diabetes in Qatar is peer-to-peer patient education. This will ensure that patients who are facing challenges from diabetes share their experiences (Khoja et al., 2010). As a result, disease awareness strategies will receive a significant boost leading the establishment of well controlled diabetes environment.

Moreover, establishment of specialized diabetes centers across the nation for better diabetes care will enhance diabetes treatment and management through the provision of education and training for diabetic patients.

Conclusion

In a brief conclusion, Qatar is facing an enormous public healthcare challenge caused by the high prevalence rates of diabetes. In the past decade, prevalence rates for diabetes have more than doubled because the country had inefficient healthcare system. The country faces several health inequalities which have contributed significantly to the raising prevalence trends of diabetes among its population. For instance, social determinants of health such as education, informal sector employment and urbanization have barred Qatar's healthcare system from realizing remarkable success in controlling diabetes. Moreover, lack of reliable health policy is believed to be one of the most significant factors which have increased diabetes disease burden in Qatar. However, the country is in the process of designing an integrated healthcare system to enhance preventive care through public health governance.

References

Al-Maadheed, G. & Qahtani, A. (2011). *National Health Strategy 2011-2016*. Retrieved from http://www.qu.edu.qa/pharmacy/components/upcoming_events_material/Qatar_National_Health_Strategy.pdf

ANSA. (2013). *Qatar: Surge in Diabetes/Obesity, Unhealthy Arab Habits*. Retrieved from http://www.ansamed.info/ansamed/en/news/sections/generalnews/2012/03/13/visualizza_new.html_131156617.html

Bener, A. et al. (2009). Prevalence of Diagnosed and Undiagnosed Diabetes Mellitus and Its Risk Factors in a Population-Based Study of Qatar. *Diabetes Research and Clinical Practice*, 84(1):99–106.

Brandt, A. & Churchill, L. (2003). *Bittersweet: Diabetes, Insulin, and the Transformation of Illness*. Chapel Hill, NC: University of North Carolina Press.

Center for Disease Control and Prevention (2010). *Diabetes Research and Statistics*. Retrieved 5 March. 2012. http://www.cdc.gov/diabetes/consumer/research.htm

Coddington, D. & Hisnanick, J. (2001). Clinical Characteristics of Non-insulin-dependent Diabetes Mellitus among Southwestern American Indian Youths. *Journal of Health, Population and Nutrition*, 19: 3-17.

Dwevedi, A. & Goyal, M. (2010). *Diabetes Rate Alarmingly High in Qatar*. Retrieved from http://www.thepeninsulaqatar.com/qatar/119521-diabetes-rate-alarmingly-high-in-qatar.html

Khoja, T. et al. (2010). *Diabetes: The Hidden Pandemic and Its Impact on the Middle East and Northern Africa*. Brussels, Belgium: International Diabetes Federation. Retrieved from http://www.novonordisk.com/images/about_us/changing-diabetes/PDF/Leadership%20forum%20pdfs/MENA%20Forum/MENA_Diabetes_briefing_book_EN.pdf

Masharani, U. (2008). *Diabetes Demystified*. New York, NY: McGraw-Hill.

Pompei, P. (2006). Diabetes Mellitus in Later Life. *Generations*, 30: 5-14.

Siddiqi, S. & Watts, S. (2008). *Social Determinants of Health in the Eastern Mediterranean Region*. Retrieved from http://gis.emro.who.int/HealthSystemObservatory/Workshops/QatarConference/PPt%20converted%20to%20PDF/Day%203/SDH%20and%20Health%20Equity/Dr%20Sameen%20Siddiqi%20and%20Susan%20Watts%20-%20Social%20Determinants%20of%20Health.pdf

YOUR KNOWLEDGE HAS VALUE

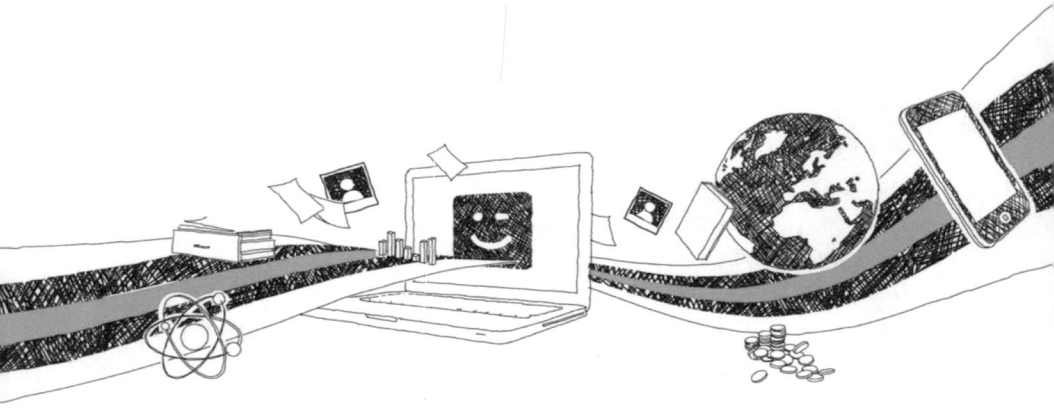

- We will publish your bachelor's and master's thesis, essays and papers

- Your own eBook and book - sold worldwide in all relevant shops

- Earn money with each sale

Upload your text at www.GRIN.com
and publish for free

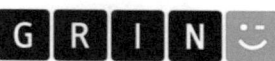